# Weight Loss Guide for Beginners

## *How to Lose Weight Fast to Optimize Your Health, Revitalize Your Appearance & Rapidly Increase Your Energy*

*Elizabeth Ryan*

# Table of Contents

# Introduction

I want to thank you and congratulate you for purchasing this book!

This book contains proven steps and strategies on how to lose weight in 5 easy steps!

Many people, adults and teens alike, are suffering from obesity and being overweight. These are conditions that have become more and more common over the years due to the advent of fast food and high technology. Though these factors only want nothing else but to deliver comfort to you, the consumer, there are still unexpected effects that may come out of them. Young children get more and more obese primarily because of the foods they eat and the type of lifestyle they have. Because of this, being overweight and obese have stopped being just aesthetic concerns; they have become a worldwide health burden. One of the interventions used in decreasing the incidence of overweight and obesity, and in decreasing the incidence of their complications, is the utilization of weight loss programs. This ebook will guide you through how to lose weight in the safest and fastest way!

Thanks again for purchasing this book, I hope you enjoy it! Please take some time to stop by and LIKE our Facebook page:

https://www.facebook.com/joypublishing


With gratitude,

Elizabeth Ryan

# Chapter 1

## Why Lose Weight Now?

In recent years, the incidence of obesity has been steadily, if not logarithmically, rising. A survey conducted in 2008 revealed that about 35% of adults in the world are overweight, and about 11% are obese. And until recently, the statistics have shown an increasing trend of obesity among the younger population, most especially those belonging in the age of puberty.

Being weight and obese are now becoming global burdens. These two conditions have been associated with a lot of diseases, such as cardiovascular disorders and Diabetes Mellitus, which are included in the 10 leading causes of morbidity and mortality in the world. Overweight and obese people should not only be concerned about their figure or their physical appearance but they should also be concerned about their health.

There are many health problems associated with being overweight and obese since many organs are negatively affected by these two conditions. The respiratory, cardiovascular, reproductive and the metabolic systems can all be affected. How do these two conditions affect these body systems?

Have you ever seen a young obese man run for a few seconds and then get short of breath immediately afterwards? This is a rather common scenario that you could have already seen or experienced. Obese and overweight people sometimes experience shortness of breath after doing a light activity because of the following reasons: 1) Their thorax is being compressed by fats, hence limiting lung expansion; and 2) they get tired easily because of their slow metabolism and because of their weight. They would usually stop halfway while going up the stairs or they do not usually finish one whole lap when they jog.

The cardiovascular and metabolic systems are two systems that are predominantly affected by obesity. There is a higher risk for development of atherosclerosis and heart attack in obese people. This is attributed to the excessive amounts of fats present, not only in the storage sites of adipose tissues, but also in the blood vessels, predisposing these vessels to occlusion. Once cholesterol molecules have accumulated inside the walls of these arteries and veins, there will be subsequent decrease in blood flow that can lead to heart attack. The metabolic system, on the other hand, is affected because the metabolic rate decreases as the body's fat content increases. This explains why an obese person gets tired easily.

You might have been surprised when you read that the reproductive system is actually affected. It may sound weird to you, but it is true. Fats can cover a woman's ovaries and this may impede the release of egg cells out into the fallopian tube. This is the reason why some obese women experience difficulties in conceiving children. As a result, the sperm reaches an empty fallopian tube and dies soon thereafter. Women may also experience amenorrhea, or the lack of menses, or anovulation, or lack of ovulation. Some may have menorrhagia or metrorrhagia, two conditions that are characterized either by an increase in the frequency or duration of menses.

Because of the many diseases that are associated with obesity, it is but important to keep a physically fit body and a weight that is appropriate for one's stature and age. Losing weight will not just keep you away from these diseases, but will also surely make you feel good about yourself, make you look and feel younger, and also give you your energy back! Read on to know the *5-step weight loss plan*!

# Chapter 2

# Step 1: Know How Much You Need to Lose

Losing weight is not just a simple goal. Before you step onto your treadmill or grab a bite of your green leafy vegetables, you have to know first how much you need to lose. In other words, you have to know which is normal and which is not to determine whether you are on the right track or going the opposite way.

Many people would simply base their progress on their weight. A 10-lb decrease in their weight would already be seen as a success and so they would stop there. Of course, weight is primary in this kind of plan, but there are other things that people have to consider.

Being overweight is defined as having a body mass index of 25 to 29.9, while obesity is defined as having a body mass index or BMI of 30 or more. Obesity is further classified into two types: Type 1 and Type 2 obesity. Type 1 Obesity is defined as having a BMI of 30 to 34.9, while 35 and above for the second type. BMI is the ratio of your weight in kilograms (kg) over your height in meters squared ($m^2$). For example, you are currently weighing 80 kg and your height is 160 cm. To convert your height to $m^2$, you simply need to divide 160 by 100 and square the answer.

**Example:** 160 cm/ 100= (1.6 m)$^2$= **2.56 m$^2$**

**BMI**= 80 kg/2.56= **31.25**

**Interpretation:** Obese

Now that you know how to determine whether you are obese or not, you also have to know whether or not you have reached your goal by comparing it with the normal values. A BMI of 20 to 24.9 is the expected normal value. A BMI falling below this range indicates that the person is underweight.

For example, your weight before starting on your weight loss program was 80 kg. Now, after three weeks of continuous dieting and training, you have found out that you have lost 10 kg! To determine whether you have succeeded in achieving your goal or not, then you should compute for your BMI.

**BMI** = 70 kg/2.56 = 27.34

**Interpretation:** Overweight

From obesity, you have managed to lose some weight and are now considered overweight. This may be considered good news but remember that overweight is still not healthy. You decided to go on with your weight loss program until you lost another 10 kg after three more weeks. So now, you have to compute your BMI again.

**BMI** = 60 kg/ 2.56 = 23.43

**Interpretation:** *Normal*

How rewarding would it be to get your BMI back to normal, right? After six weeks of a little bit of sacrifice, you finally managed to achieve your goal! Imagine going through those six weeks without getting a hint whether you were making progress or not. Knowing how much you need to lose should not discourage you from losing weight; rather, it should challenge you to get your health back without any hesitation. Take this first step and you won't get lost in your weight loss journey.

# Chapter 3

## Step 2: Start Walking

Walking 10,000 steps a day is not just ideal for preventing the onset of cardiovascular problems, but it is also a good practice to help you lose weight. After knowing how much you need to lose, you can officially start your weight loss program by walking for a longer period of time or for a greater distance.

Walking is a simple yet a very effective way of losing weight. It might seem like a very light activity as if there is nothing much going on inside your body when you walk, but walking actually mobilizes your fats and stimulates your other organs to work. This is the reason why walking has been associated with a lot of health benefits.

One of the health benefits of walking is that it allows your liver to metabolize your fats instead of just letting your cholesterol stay inside your tissues. The fats that are stored in the adipose tissues of your belly, thighs and arms are broken down into fatty acids that will be used for the production of energy which ultimately leads to your weight loss.

Walking also improves your blood circulation, delivering much of the nutrients and oxygen to the different body parts. You might even notice a glow in your skin after walking for some time as a result of an increase in blood flow. The improvement in your circulation is further augmented by the pumping actions of the muscles in your lower extremities—actions that are strengthened by walking and other physical activities. Your muscle pump helps your heart in pushing the blood to different parts of the body and improves your venous return. An adequate venous return helps in maintaining normal blood pressure.

Most people would say that they don't have the time to walk, but what they don't know is that they can actually incorporate walking into their daily activities, even if they are just sitting in front of their desks or are busy with their work. Have you heard of treadmill desks? These are desks that have built-in treadmill bases. You just have to control the speed of the treadmill to prevent dizziness after using it.

There are other ways by which you can increase your physical activity. Here are some of them:

1. **Do not use the remote control.** Technology can really make one's life as comfortable as it can be. Recently-released televisions even have motion and voice sensors so you won't even have to grab the remote control. You will just have to say what you want the appliance to do and it will do precisely that. Motion sensors will also detect your movement and will respond according to the action you've made. You can now do a lot of things with just a snap of a finger. However, you have to remember that too much comfort is dangerous. People who have been used to using a remote control would not want to move anymore. They just want to lie down on their beds or stay seated on their soft couches, not thinking that they are letting their fats hide under their skin. What you can do is to forget that you have a remote control and walk towards

your TV to change the channel turn up the volume. A few steps would not hurt and would actually make a lot of difference.

2.  **Walk your way to school, work or to the grocery store.** If you have a lot of time to do some grocery shopping or if you leave for school or work early, then you can just walk instead of driving your car. If your short on time, you can ride your bicycle.

3.  **Use the stairs.** If you are going up a floor or two, then using the stairs would be a better choice than using the elevator or escalator. You can already burn a considerable number of calories by just walking up a flight of stairs.

# Chapter 4

## Step 3: Avoid Foods That Can Make You Gain Weight

In this day and age, there are already a lot of foods that can make you gain extra pounds. What are the foods that you have to avoid? Basically, the foods that you have to avoid are those that are rich in fats, especially saturated fats, sugar and carbohydrates. Foods that are rich in saturated fats are dairy products, beef, pork, and lard. You have to take note that even lean meats contain fats.

We can easily order fatty burgers, oily and salty french fries, ice cream, pasta, flavored coffee topped with a cholesterol-rich whip cream, sinfully sweet desserts, and a lot more. Don't they seem irresistible and tempting? But wait, there is the catch: they are full of sugar, fats and starches that can make you gain those unwanted pounds.

Losing weight is largely a sacrifice. You have to do something you do not usually do and you cannot eat what you want to eat. Ironic, isn't it? Cutting down on your favorite foods might just be the biggest factor hindering you from taking that one step forward towards good health. You might be imagining yourself munching on that slice of chocolate cake or joyfully sipping that cup of coffee complete with a caramel topping and whip cream!

This step is actually one of the greatest challenges that people encounter when they try to lose weight. Some people who are trying to lose weight cannot let go of these foods and fail the program while some just do not enter the program at all. How do we make this step bearable and successful?

Cutting down on your favorite foods does not have to be sudden. Here are some things that you can do to overcome this challenge:

- If you are used to indulging on heavenly desserts after breakfast, lunch and dinner, then you can probably cut down one of them or decrease their amount gradually. For example, if you usually eat a whole bar of milk chocolate after eating, what you can do is to divide the bar into two: eat the first half during breakfast and the other half after lunch. If you can sacrifice eating dessert after dinner, the better.

- Use an imaginary line to divide your plate into four: the first part is for protein sources, such as meat and fish; the second and third parts are for vegetables and fruits; the fourth part is for your grains or pasta. This helps you control the types of food that you eat.

- Before going to the grocery store for some shopping, make a list of the food that you have to buy. This guides you in prioritizing what you should and should not eat. This will also keep you from going into that part of the grocery where you can find those irresistible foods. You may also want to avoid going near your favorite restaurants and coffee and pastry shops. This helps decrease the temptation.

- Eat regularly. You do not want to get hungry because it could make you eat more than what you are supposed to. You may also want to eat a light snack before leaving the house to give you enough energy to do what you need to do without needing to take a side trip to a fast food nearby.

# Chapter 5

## Step 4:  Indulge On Foods That Can Make You Lose Weight

Losing weight is not simply about cutting down on your food intake or sacrificing the food that you want to eat. It is also about eating more of the foods that can make you lose weight. These foods can decrease the levels of cholesterol in your blood, remove toxins inside your body, and boost your metabolism.

Here are some of the foods that you should have in your kitchen right now:

### 1. Oatmeal

Many people do not want oatmeal because it tastes so "plain," but what they do not know is that oatmeal is actually very healthy for the body. It is rich in fiber that promotes good digestion and helps decrease blood cholesterol levels. Oatmeal is also enriched with vitamins and minerals hence making it a healthy choice!

Fiber causes a decrease in blood levels of cholesterol by facilitating their elimination. Insoluble fiber binds with bile and eliminates it through the stool. Bile is a fat emulsifier produced by the liver. What is surprising about bile is that it is actually made up of cholesterol. Hence, eliminating bile would also mean eliminating cholesterol. When the liver senses that the levels of bile are decreasing, it would mobilize the cholesterol molecules present in your body tissues and use them to synthesize more bile.

If you want your oatmeal to be just as tasty as your other breakfast meals, you can actually add some slices of banana and apple into your meal. You may also opt to use non-fat milk for your oatmeal. Expect to feel full easily and for a longer time with oatmeal.

## 2.  Buckwheat pasta

If you love pasta but are currently on a diet, then you can try this pasta out! Buckwheat pasta would make a healthy alternative for your spaghetti noodles because they are rich in protein, unlike the usual pastas that are rich in carbohydrates and starches.

## 3. Yogurt

Why indulge in fatty and sugary ice cream when you can have healthy yogurt? You can actually experiment with yogurt by mixing different kinds of fruits or by using it as a substitute if you are cooking a dish that needs some dairy product. You can substitute yogurt for mayonnaise or all-purpose cream. Yogurt is low in fat so you don't have to worry about your blood cholesterol levels afterwards.

## 4. Salmon, Tuna, Mackerel and Sardines

Speaking of fats, salmon, tuna, mackerel and sardines are rich in a fatty acid called Omega-3. This is something that you might have already heard or seen from an advertisement. What makes Omega-3 different from the other fats? Omega-3 fatty acid is a type of an unsaturated fatty acid. Remember that it is the saturated type of fat that is unhealthy. Unsaturated fats, unlike the saturated ones, get broken down or emulsified easily and do not form into solid masses under body temperature. Hence, these fats do not form plugs inside your blood vessels, a characteristic that is consistent with the saturated fats. Omega-3 fatty acids also have anti-inflammatory properties, which may be helpful among people who have a hyperactive immune system. Remember to include these Omega-3 rich fish in your grocery list.

## 5. Avocado

If salmon, tuna, mackerel, and sardines are rich in omega-3, avocado, on the other hand, is rich in HDL. High density lipoprotein or HDL is a type of cholesterol that carries fats from the tissues back to the liver for their degradation. HDL has been called the good cholesterol for this reason. It is also because of this fat content why avocado seems to increase your satiety.

## 6. Wheat Bread

Breads are just perfect for anything- breakfast, snacks, lunch or dinner, and it would be a shame if you are going to totally eliminate bread from your diet. Instead of the usual white bread that you eat, you can give wheat bread a try. Wheat is rich in fiber, helping you eliminate cholesterol, while at the same time detoxifying and cleansing your gastrointestinal tract, and increasing your satiety. Eat it with some lettuce, tomatoes and fish fillet, instead of the usual burger patty. It would definitely taste just as awesome!

Here are three recipes that you can try at home:

# A. Grilled Salmon with Avocado

*Ingredients:*

- 1 lb salmon fillet
- Salt and pepper
- 1 tbsp fresh lemon juice
- 2 tbsp soy sauce
- 1 tsp chopped basil
- 1 avocado

*Procedure:*

1. Marinate the salmon fillet in lemon juice, basil, soy sauce, salt and pepper for at least an hour.
2. Grill the salmon over low fire.
3. Serve with avocados.

### B. Tuna Salad

*Ingredients:*

- 1 canned tuna, drained
- 1 tbsp chopped peanuts
- Lettuce
- 1 tomato, sliced in circles
- 1 small onion, finely chopped
- 1 tbsp pineapple juice
- Parmesan cheese to top

*Procedure:*

1. Layer lettuce and tomatoes on a plate.
2. In a small bowl, mix pineapple juice and canned tuna.
3. Top this mixture onto the lettuce and tomatoes.
4. Top with onions, peanuts, and cheese.
5. Serve and enjoy!

## C. Fish Fillet Sandwich

*Ingredients:*

- 2 slices wheat bread
- ¼ lb cream dory fillet
- 1 egg
- ½ cup bread crumbs
- Lettuce and tomatoes
- 3 tbsp canola oil

*Procedure:*

1. Beat the egg in a small bowl.
2. Dip cream dory fillet into the beaten egg.
3. Roll the fillet over the breadcrumbs.
4. Fry in canola oil over low heat until golden brown.
5. Assemble the sandwich. Top lettuce, tomatoes and fish fillet over the bread then serve.

# Chapter 6

## Step 5: Develop your Exercise Habit

Just like walking, exercise has a lot of health benefits. Aside from mobilizing your fat stores, exercise is also known for its feel-good effect. Have you ever experienced feeling down and then suddenly getting amped up after some dancing or doing some exercise routines? That is because exercise stimulates the release of your endogenous opioids, also called endorphins and enkephalins. These are chemicals produced by the brain that bind to opioid receptors, thus giving you that feeling of elation.

Exercise also improves the function of insulin. This is a hormone produced by the pancreas to lower blood glucose levels. Insulin is secreted in a basal level; however, in the presence of increased blood glucose, as in after a high-glucose meal, insulin is secreted in greater numbers. In certain conditions like Diabetes Mellitus or DM, there is either insulin resistance or a decrease in the production of insulin. Insulin resistance refers to that state of the cells wherein they do not respond to the effects of insulin anymore. The glucose remains in the blood instead of being taken up by these cells. This is the main reason why exercise is being recommended as part of lifestyle modification techniques among diabetic patients.

Here are some exercises that can make you lose weight in no time:

## 1. Dancing

You might be expecting some weight-lifting or a treadmill run in this case, but the problem with those routines is that once you stop doing them, your fats would seem to wake up from a deep slumber and cause you to gain your weight again. Dancing is a good alternative for these exercises because of the following reasons: 1) Your whole body moves, making weight loss easier; 2) Depending on the part of the body that you usually use, dancing can tone your muscles and shape your waist up. 3) It is a fun way of losing weight. Instead of counting how many times you have raised that dumbbell, you can just go along with the music, feel the rhythm, and forget all about counting.

## 2. Cardio Exercises

One of the most effective warm-up and weight-losing activities is a cardio exercise. They can range from simple walking, to running, or jumping. One cardio exercise that will surely make you lose weight is jumping using a skipping rope. Don't get discouraged by the exhausting nature of jumping because it just means that you are getting the results that you are expecting. What you can do is to jump with both of your legs using a jumping rope for 30 seconds every 30 second-interval. This means that a set is equal to 1 minute- 30 seconds jumping and 30 seconds resting. Do 12 sets. If you are a beginner, you can start with 6 sets first and then increase the number of sets by an increment of two every 3 days.

### 3. Part-specific Exercises

There are times when only a part of your body gets to lose fat while some parts retain theirs. To avoid this, you can perform some focused exercises. If you think that your arm is too big or round for your body, then you can either plank, do some push-ups or try boxing. These exercises help you tone your muscles so that they won't look flabby when you lose weight. Thigh and leg exercises include jogging, leg extensions and squatting.

Aside from the 5 steps presented here, one must also know how to keep track of one's progress. Always evaluate whether you are achieving your goals or not. You need to measure how much weight you have lost from the start of your program to the end to determine whether your program is working or not. Losing weight does not happen overnight. You need to be patient and committed to be able to succeed in your weight loss regimen. Good luck!

# Conclusion

Thank you again for purchasing this book!

I hope this book was able to help you to overcome your hesitation and fears in losing weight.

The next step is to take that first step and start knowing how much you need to lose!

In addition, please remember to check out our Facebook page in order to find other resources and upcoming promotions:

https://www.facebook.com/joypublishing

With sincere thanks,


Elizabeth Ryan

# One Last Thing...

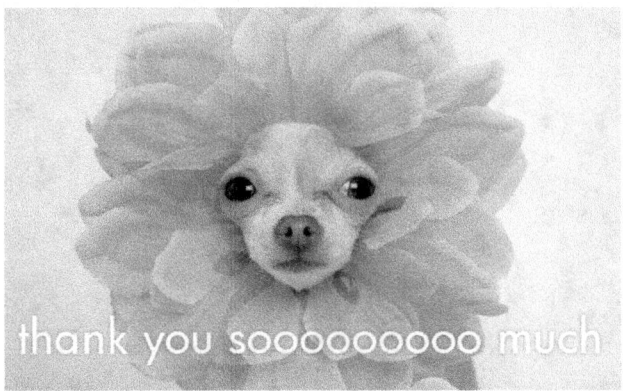

If you believe that this book is worth sharing, would you please take the time to let others know how it affected your life? If it turns out to make a difference in the lives of others, they will be forever grateful to you, as will I.

www.ingramcontent.com/pod-product-compliance
Lightning Source LLC
Chambersburg PA
CBHW061941280526
45787CB00004B/1681